YOGA FOR BEGINNERS

*Your Guide to Master Yoga Poses
while calming your mind, be stress free,
and boost your self-esteem!*

ALEXANDER YAMASHITA

YOGA FOR BEGINNERS

Copyright © 2015 by Alexander Yamashita.
All rights reserved.

This document is geared towards providing exact and reliable information in regards to the topic and issue covered. The publication is sold with the idea that the publisher is not required to render accounting, officially permitted, or otherwise, qualified services. If advice is necessary, legal or professional, a practiced individual in the profession should be ordered.

From a Declaration of Principles which was accepted and approved equally by a Committee of the American Bar Association and a Committee of Publishers and Associations.

In no way is it legal to reproduce, duplicate, or transmit any part of this document in either electronic means or in printed format. Recording of this publication is strictly prohibited and any storage of this document is not allowed unless with written permission from the publisher. All rights reserved.

The information provided herein is stated to be truthful and consistent, in that any liability, in terms of inattention or otherwise, by any usage or abuse of any policies, processes, or directions contained within is the solitary and utter responsibility of the recipient reader. Under no circumstances will any legal responsibility or blame be held against the publisher for any reparation, damages, or monetary loss due to the information herein, either directly or indirectly.

Respective authors own all copyrights not held by the publisher.

The information herein is offered for informational purposes solely, and is universal as so. The presentation of the information is without contract or any type of guarantee assurance.

The trademarks that are used are without any consent, and the publication of the trademark is without permission or backing by the trademark owner. All trademarks and brands within this book are for clarifying purposes only and are the owned by the owners themselves, not affiliated with this document.

TABLE OF CONTENTS

Introduction 4
Chapter 1: Yoga and All that You Need to Know before practicing it 6
Chapter 2: Basic Poses often used in Yoga and How to Do it 12
Chapter 3: Warm-up Routines for Yoga 29
Chapter 4: Basic Routines 35
Chapter 5: Preparing for the Advanced Yoga Poses 42
Chapter 6: The Yoga Diet 50
Preview Of 'Zen for Beginners' 53
Check Out My Other Books 65
Conclusion 66

INTRODUCTION

I want to thank you and congratulate you for downloading the book, *Yoga for Beginners: Your Guide to Master Yoga Poses while calming your mind, be stress free, and boost your self-esteem!*

Yoga is a belief that a man's mind, body and spirit should work in harmony with the environment and his own self. To achieve this, his emotions, actions and intelligence should all be in balance.

Most people nowadays are more interested in yoga as a form of exercise. Many are practicing yoga because it is proven to help calm the mind, reduce stress, relieve pain, and lose weight (which most often translates to an increase in confidence). As a matter of fact, many doctors now accept its therapeutic benefits as they've seen it do wonders on their own patients.

Some who are not familiar with yoga think that it is an exercise composed of poses that are also impossible to do. This is why some people become rather hesitant about practicing it, or even trying it. Though it may be true that some poses require impressive flexibility, there are many poses that can be done by beginners or those who are still inflexible.

With this book, you will learn everything about how to begin practicing Yoga. It will teach you some basic techniques on how to prepare your body, mind, and spirit. It will teach also teach you how to slowly achieve the flexibility needed for advanced poses – in a safe, gradual way (rushing things won't be beneficial in this kind of self-improvement pursuit as doing so will only lead to injury).

The book will also include basic sequences of poses, which you can use to create an exercise routine. You'll also discover what you need to learn about the essentials of yoga.

In other words, you'll know exactly what you should prepare (such as mats and straps) before starting a healing exercise that can help you achieve a balanced and calm mind, spirit, and body. In addition, you will know the proper attire for doing yoga – the sort of clothes that you'll be able to move in.

If you're worried that you'll only get to read about beginner-level poses and routines, you will be glad to know that this book also serves as a preview on the more advanced side of yoga. After all, most beginners eventually yearn to try something more challenging. To achieve a proper balance between enthusiasm and safety, several tips are also provided for those aiming to become advanced yoga practitioners.

As you might have heard, diet is also an important aspect of this mind-calming, stress-reducing, and confidence-boosting endeavor. That's why this book also features an entire chapter dedicated to proper yoga nutrition. It won't be strict diet though, as you will only be taught how to food items that could help you reach your goal. Of course, that also means you'll become more familiar with those that won't do you any good.

Thanks again for purchasing this book,
I hope you enjoy it!
Alexander Yamashita

CHAPTER 1:
YOGA AND ALL THAT YOU NEED TO KNOW BEFORE PRACTICING IT

Yoga is a practice that originated in India. It was discovered 500 years ago. It was developed to show the appreciation for the body. Ancient yogis believed that the body should be treated well and respected because it is the main medium for man's growth and work.

Yoga has six forms. These are breathing, meditation, exercise, devotion, self-control and service.

Most yogis, however, often follow only the three main forms of yoga which are breathing, meditation and exercise. These three forms are incorporated in what is known as Hatha Yoga.

Hatha Yoga
Hatha yoga is the most popular branch of yoga, especially in Western countries. It is usually perceived as an exercise which involves twisting and difficult posture, but it is more than just an exercise.

Hatha Yoga is regarded as the therapeutic branch of yoga. The main purpose of this branch is to achieve total wellness of the body and to gain a peaceful mind. Some yoga experts even claim that a ninety minute session of yoga per week can already do many wonders on one's health.

Each pose of Hatha Yoga has different health benefits. Below are some of the common health benefits you can get from practicing yoga.

1. It tones the muscles.
2. It helps the yogi sleep better.
3. It relieves muscle pains, muscle injuries and migraine.
4. It improves blood circulation.
5. It improves the respiratory health of the yogi.
6. It improves the digestive health of the yogi.
7. It boosts the body's immunity.
8. It helps control the appetite and aids in losing weight.
9. It improves sexual performance.
10. It decreases stress.

There are six main types of Hatha Yoga. This book will focus more on the techniques and poses that are easy to follow, but will still let you achieve a peaceful mind and a healthy body.

Yogi refers to the person who practices any form of yoga.

Essential Equipment for Yoga

Before going to a yoga class or trying yoga on your own at home, make sure that you have the basic equipment. Below is the list of the things you may need during a yoga session.

1. Yoga Mat

A yoga mat may not be essential if you are doing yoga at home, but it can help a lot in your routines. The mat will help you define the space you need for each pose. It also provides as a flat cushion for your body, considering that you would be doing some poses on the floor. The mat will also prevent you from slipping, especially in doing feet-spreading techniques.

The standard size for a yoga mat is 24-inch by 68-inch. Yoga mats tend to be slippery at the beginning. You may wash it hard and let it dry thoroughly to make it non-slippery or you could just wear it out.

2. Yoga outfits
For beginners, yoga can be a bit discomforting. This is why many experts suggest that you should wear outfits that you are comfortable with. However, you also have to consider your flexibility.

For women, a sleeveless tank top and leggings are ideal yoga outfits. For men, sleeveless shirts and sweatpants are ideal. Just make sure that the tops are fitted to your body or it may slip up while you are doing your routine.

3. Blankets
Blankets are good substitutes for the mats when you have to do poses where you need to lie down or spread your body wide.

4. Straps
Straps are used as your extensions for your hands if you cannot reach another part of your body.

5. Bricks or Pillows
Bricks or pillows work as the floor extension if you cannot reach the floor in some poses. You can also use thick books or magazines.

6. Towels
Yoga exercises can make you sweat a lot. You have to use them to wipe your sweat. Towels can also be used as straps.

The Do's and Don'ts Before, During, and After Yoga Exercise
Here are the things you should do or should not do before, during, and after yoga exercise or class.

Things you should do:
1. Hydrate yourself. Drink a lot of water before and after the exercise.

2. Familiarize yourself with the basic yoga poses. Though it will be taught by your teacher if you take a yoga class, it will help you become more comfortable if you have an idea about how to do basic poses.
3. Do not be afraid to ask help. If you have poses that you cannot do on your own, ask the teacher or a fellow yogi for some help.

Things you should not do:
1. Do not eat heavy meals before the yoga exercise. Just have a few pieces of saltine crackers an hour before the exercise. Save the big meal after the exercise.
2. Do not drink a lot of water during the yoga session. If you get thirsty during the exercise, just take a few sips to moisten your mouth and throat.
3. Do not wear shoes or socks. Wearing shoes can make your feet heavy when doing some poses, while socks may make you slip from the floor or mat when doing the poses.
4. Do not be absent-minded. You have to clear your mind when you do yoga exercises, but you do not have to leave your mind blank. You need to have an active mind to maintain our coordination with your body.

How to avoid Yoga Injuries
Even the basic poses of yoga can cause injury to the body if done in a wrong way. Thus, it is important that the yogi should know his limits and arm himself with knowledge in order to avoid yoga injuries.

Here are some yoga injuries you have to watch out for when doing yoga:
1. *Back injuries.* Back sprains are common during yoga practice. This is because yogis tend to overstretch their lower back ligaments during the stretching poses. What you should be careful of is your spine disc. Wrong or improper twists can badly damage

your disc and can cause extreme back pain.
2. Wrists injuries. The wrists are likely to be sprained when doing poses that uses your hand as support. It usually happens when the hands were improperly placed and could not support the body's weight. It is suggested that if you have weak wrists, you should learn to shift the weight of your body away from it.
3. Neck injuries. The most common injury in the neck is the overstretched nape. Many yogis usually pull their head back to stretch their front necks during the poses, but they usually forgot the back of the neck. So, when they need to press their chin on their chest, their nape is sprained.
4. Dizziness and lightheadedness. Though this is not an actual injury, many yogis suffer from dizziness and lightheadedness when doing yoga workout. This is usually caused by lack of hydration and lack of eyes and breathing warm-up.

Here are some safety tips during yoga practice:
1. Do the proper warm-up. Many injuries, such as pulled ligaments and sprains, happen because the yogi did not do a proper warm-up routine. This book will give you a number of proper routines that will help you during your practice.
2. Do not force yourself. If your feet cannot touch your head or your body cannot bend so low, just stop where your limit takes you. Let your flexibility develop slowly.
3. Do not do yoga when you have injuries. Yoga is used as a therapy to strengthen the muscles and the joints, but it is not recommended to people with injuries. If you have joint injuries, back pains or health concerns, you should ask your yoga instructor or physician first before taking on any of the yoga poses.
4. Ask for help from a reputable instructor or expert yogi. Though the basic poses of yoga are easy to

execute, it is still recommended that you ask the help of reputable instructor or expert yogi. They may help you advance faster and can help you practice safely. It is recommended that before taking on yoga on your own, you should at least attend a basic class so you would know the safety measures you have to observe when doing poses.

5. Avoid showing off or competing with others. You should remember that you are doing the yoga for yourself and not to show off or compete with friends or other yogis. If you use yoga to show off, you won't be able to calm your mind and you'll defeat the purpose of doing yoga.
6. When doing yoga on your own, be sure that someone is with you or there are people nearby so that someone can immediately help you when you accidentally injured yourself during the practice.

Now that you know what you need and how to be safe when doing a yoga practice, you are ready to do some basic yoga poses and routines.

Just remember to mind your safety first before trying any of the poses.

CHAPTER 2:
BASIC POSES OFTEN USED IN YOGA AND HOW TO DO IT

Many are hesitant about practicing yoga not just because it appears to be painful and uncomfortable, but also because it involves a lot of poses.

Yogis usually have to do a number of poses to complete an exercise routine. Some people may think that memorizing the poses and the sequence can be tough. What they do not know is that these poses are only varieties of ten basic poses.

Below are the basic poses often used in yoga routines and the steps on how to do them.

1. Easy pose. This is usually the first pose in Asanas Yoga or Sitting Yoga. It is a typical meditation pose.

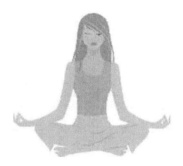

How to do it:
- Sit on the floor or on the mat.
- Cross your legs. Place your feet below your knees.
- Place your hands on your knees.
- Straighten your head and body.
- Inhale for five seconds. Hold your breath for three seconds. Exhale for eight seconds. Repeat the breathing five more times.

How to safely transition to a different pose from the Easy Pose:
- Straighten your legs. Rotate your feet four times in a clockwise direction and then four times in a counter-clockwise direction.
- Stretch your legs and feet for five seconds.
- Shake your legs a little before doing a different pose.

Tips for beginners:
- If you find it difficult to sit flat on the floor or on the mat, you may use a thin pillow or cushion until your posture improves. You may try doing it on your couch for a while until you are ready to do it on the ground.
- If you find it difficult to straighten your back, you can do the easy pose with your back pressed on a flat wall. If you have a partner, you can do this pose while sitting back to back.

Health or Therapeutic Benefits of Easy Pose
- It helps you breathe normally.
- It relieves back pains and stiff necks or muscles.
- It improves the colon and the digestive system.
- It helps relieve heart burns and acid reflux.

2. The Mountain Pose. This is the template of most yoga standing poses. This is also the basic pose for the breathing exercise and the starting pose for the Sun Salutation routine. It is similar to yawning while standing up and while the hands are on the side.

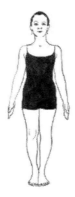

How to do it:
- Stand straight with your feet together. Close your eyes.
- Place your hands on the sides. Keep your fingers together.
- Inhale for five seconds. Hold your breath for three seconds. Exhale for eight seconds.
- Then raise your hands up towards the sky. Stretch your arms up.
- Lift your heels up and stand on your tiptoes.
- Inhale for five seconds. Hold your breath for three seconds. Exhale for eight seconds while moving your arms and heels down.
- Repeat the process five more times.

Tips for beginners:
- If you find it difficult to stand with your feet together, you can spread it a little to gain balance. Try to make your feet closer for the next session.

Health or Therapeutic Benefits of the Mountain Pose
- It helps you breathe normally.
- It calms your nerves.
- It improves the standing posture and improves the height.
- It improves focus and balance.
- It tones the arm and leg muscles.
- It removes sleepiness.

3. The Tree Pose. This is one of the pose which you can shift from the mountain position. It is also known as the balancing pose. It is called the tree pose because the posture of the yogi is comparable to a sturdy tree.

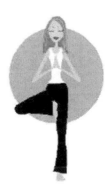

How to do it:
- Stand in the basic mountain pose.
- Slowly raise your left foot and place it on your right thigh. The toes should be pointing towards the floor.
- While standing on your right leg, slowly join your palms together above your head.
- Reach up as far as you can. Take a deep breath. Hold the position as long as you can.
- Slowly release your breath as you lower your hands back to the sides.
- Repeat the process on the other foot. Do three or four sets for each routine.

Tips for beginners
- If you find it difficult to place your feet on your thighs, you can start by just placing them on your calves. Just raise the position of your feet a bit higher every session.
- If you find it difficult to balance on one leg while raising your hands, you can just place your hands on your chest. This is called the praying pose.
- If you cannot stand on one leg, you can stand next to a chair or to the wall to help with your balance.

Health Benefits of Tree Pose
- It strengthens the knees, thighs, calves and the spine.
- It improves the posture and the balance, especially of those with flat feet.
- It improves the concentration.

4. The Warrior pose. This is another transition from the mountain pose. It usually follows the tree position. The warrior pose has three parts. The first part is to strengthen of the middle section of the body. The second part is to strengthen the upper body. The third part is to strengthen the lower body.

How to do it:
Basic Warrior Pose

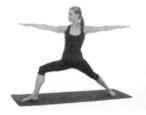

- Stand in the basic mountain pose. Twist your left feet to the side to make your feet perpendicular with each other.
- Slowly slide your left foot to the back while lowering your upper body. Your right thigh should be parallel to the floor.
- Spread your hands on a straight line. Your shoulders should align with the direction of your right knee and left heel.
- Stay in the position while taking three deep breaths.

Warrior Pose 1
- While taking another deep breath, twist your body to the right. Twist as far as possible. Exhale. Take another deep breath and return to the basic warrior pose. Exhale.
- Take another deep breath and twist your body to the left. Exhale. Take another deep breath and return to the basic warrior pose.
- While taking a deep breath, slide your left foot beside the right foot and assume the mountain pose again.
- Repeat the process with your other leg.

Warrior Pose 2

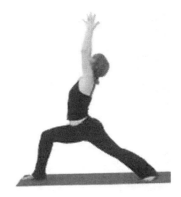

- Assume the basic warrior pose.
- Take a deep breath and join your hands above your head. Stretch your hands as high as possible. Push your hips lower to stretch your spine.
- Take three to four deep breaths. On your last exhale, slowly lower your hands and assume the basic warrior pose again.
- Return to the mountain pose.
- Repeat the process on your other leg. Repeat the process at least four times for both legs.

Warrior Pose 3

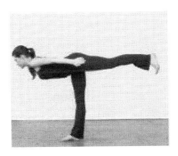

- Assume the mountain pose.
- Slip your left leg to the back.

- Take a deep breath and raise your left leg up while bending your upper body forward. Your upper body and left leg should be parallel to the floor. Your hands should be on your sides.
- Take at least four deep breaths.
- Slowly lower your leg and raise your upper body. Return to the mountain pose.
- Take a few deep breaths to relax your body.
- Repeat the process on the other leg. Repeat the process at least four times for both legs.

Tips for beginners:
- If your knee hurts when you take on the basic pose, you can raise your thighs higher. You do not have to parallel it to the floor on the first few sessions.
- If you find it difficult to balance your body while taking on warrior pose 3, you can place a chair on the front for support.

Health Benefits of Warrior Pose
- The basic warrior pose helps the respiratory system. It tones the thigh, calves and the arms. It also relieves back pains and stiff necks.
- Warrior pose 1 helps the digestive system. It helps the body detoxify.
- Warrior pose 2 increases heights. It also relieves the back pains. It tones the butt. It also helps in avoiding scoliosis and osteoporosis.
- Warrior pose 3 tones the leg parts and the butt. It improves blood circulation and normalizes the heartbeat.

5. The Triangle Pose. This is one of the basic standing poses of yoga. In some classes, it is incorporated as one of the routines for the warrior pose because the first part assumes the basic warrior pose.

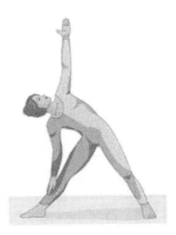

How to do it:
- Assume the mountain pose. Then, take on the basic warrior pose.
- Take a deep breath. As you exhale, bend your body to the right. Touch your ankle with your right hand. Raise your left hand up. Your fingertip and shoulder should be aligned.
- Look up and gaze at your fingers that are suspended in the air. Take at least four deep breaths. Exhale as you assume the basic warrior pose.
- Repeat the process on your left side. Repeat the pose at least four times for both sides.

Tips for the Beginners:
- If you cannot reach the ankle, just touch the shin or the calf of your leg. Or you can tie some straps around your ankles and reach for the straps instead.
- If looking up to your fingers makes you dizzy, you can look down or close your eyes instead.

Health Benefits of the Triangle Pose:
- It helps stimulate the digestive and other inner organs.
- It helps normalize sugar and blood pressure.

- It helps you avoid constipation and stimulate a good digestive system.
- It is a good therapy for people with flat feet, sciatica, osteoporosis, or scoliosis.
- It helps relieve menopausal symptoms, pre-menstrual syndromes, and dysmenorrhea.
- It helps alleviate anxiety and stress.

6. The Chair Pose. This is another standing pose.

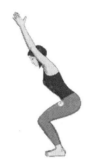

How to do it:
- Assume the mountain pose. Part your legs a little bit.
- Take a deep breath. Raise your hands above your head as you inhale. Exhale.
- Take another deep breath. Stretch your arms as far as possible as you bend your body to a 45 degree angle.
- Bend your knee and push your butt lower as you stretch your arms as far as you can.
- Take your butt deeper. Hold the position. Take a few deep breaths. Exhale as you return to the mountain pose.
- Repeat the pose at least five times.
- *Tip for the beginners:*
- If you tend to lose your balance when stretching your arm above your head, you can join them together on your chest instead.

- To guide you in the pose, place a chair at you back when doing the routine. Use the seating area of the chair as your guide as to how deep you should push your butt down.

Health Benefits of the Chair Pose
- It helps alleviate gastritis and other stomach pains caused by menstrual pains or menopausal symptoms.
- It helps relieve constipation.
- It helps tone the hip and the butt muscles.
- It improves the posture.
- It flattens the belly.

7. The Bridge Pose. This pose is the basic bending pose. Most bending poses will originate from this pose.

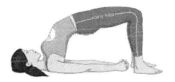

How to do it:
- Lie flat on the floor or on the mat.
- Bend your knees. Make it perpendicular with the floor.
- Place your arms on your sides. Take a deep breath.
- As you exhale, push your middle body up using the strengths from your arms and feet.
- Raise your butt as high as possible. Move your thighs so that they're parallel to the floor.
- Move your shoulders underneath your body to bend further. Join or clasp your hands under your body.
- Hold the position for at least forty seconds. Then unclasp your hands and place it again to its original position. Exhale and slowly lower your body back to the floor.
- Repeat the process at least five times.

Tip for the beginners:
- To help you start with your bend, place a pillow on your back.
- If you cannot move your thighs parallel with the floor, do not force them. Work on it slowly.

Health Benefits of the Bending Pose
- It is a therapeutic pose for people with asthma as it increases the air capacity of the lungs.
- It is a recommended therapeutic pose for those with high blood pressure, anxiety, depression, and stress.
- It alleviates insomnia and other sleep disorders.

8. The Child's pose. This is another bending pose and also, a resting pose. It is called the Child's pose because it imitates the position of a sleeping child. It is usually done after a routine so that the yogi will be energized for the next routine.

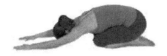

How to do it:
- Assume a kneeling position. Your thighs, knees, and feet should be joined together.
- Move your buttocks towards your heels and try to sit on them.
- Inhale and bend your body forward. As you exhale, lower your body towards your knees. Let your stomach rest on your thighs. Rest your forehead on the floor or on the mat.
- Slowly put your hands over your head. Reach as far as possible.
- Close your eyes. Hold the position for two or three minutes.
- Move your hands back to the sides and reach back as far as you can. Hold the position until you are relaxed.

- Slowly, raise your body and assume the kneeling position again.

Tips for the beginners:
- If you are still not flexible enough to have your stomach rest in your thighs or have the forehead rest on the floor, you can place a pillow to act as an extension of the floor.
- If your flab blocks your body and hinders you from assuming the position, you can raise your butt a little higher so your head can touch the floor.

Health Benefits of the Child's Pose
- It calms the mind. It is highly recommended to people with insomnia, depression and anxiety.
- It stimulates good digestion and helps in relieving bad gas from the body.
- It stretches the lower back and cures back and hip pains.
- It soothes menstrual pains.
- It prevents hernia.
- It alleviates sexual and urinary problems.

9. The Downward-Facing Dog Pose. This is one of the basic positions in yoga. It will be the starting position for different poses such as the plank pose and the locust pose.

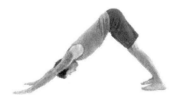

How to do it:
- Stand on your hand and knees. Your knees should be perpendicular to your hips. Your hands should be

slightly higher than your shoulders. Your back, head and buttocks should be parallel to the floor.
- Inhale. As you exhale, slowly raise your knees from the floor and shift the weight to your legs and feet.
- Take a deep breath. As you exhale, raise your hips as high as you can and tuck your head in between your arms. You should achieve an inverted letter "V" position.
- Hold the position as long as you can. Take deep breaths.
- After a few minutes, curl your knees and place it back on the floor as you exhale.
- Sit on your heels and assume the child's pose.

Tip for the beginners:
- If your hands cannot carry the weight of your upper body, you can shift the weight on your elbows.
- You may place a brick or a pillow just below your head to rest your forehead.

Health Benefits of Downward-facing Dog Pose
- It tones the arm and leg muscles.
- It improves the posture.
- It alleviates back pains and sciatica.
- It helps with blood circulation.
- It restores lost energy.

10. The Twist Poses. These are sitting yoga poses which usually follows the easy pose. They are the half-twist pose and the sage twist pose.

The Half-twist pose

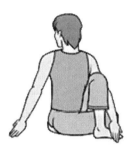

How to do it:
- From the easy pose, assume a kneeling position.
- Sit on your left feet. Raise your right leg over to the left and place your foot outside the left thighs.
- Keep your back straight. Push the heel of your right foot close to your hips or buttocks.
- Inhale. As you exhale, raise your arms at shoulder level and stretch them.
- Take a deep breath and twist to the right.
- As you exhale, bring your arms down. Place your left elbow outside the left knee.
- Inhale. Hold on to your right feet and bring your right hand to your back. As you exhale, reach your back as far as possible.
- Hold the position for as long as you can. Then, take a deep breath. As you exhale, untwist your back. Let go of your right feet and stretch your arms side to side again.
- Return to the kneeling position. Repeat the pose while sitting on your right foot.

Tips for the beginners:
- If you find it uncomfortable to sit on your feet, you can just tuck your feet close to your buttocks.
- Do the twists slowly. Do not overstretch your back.

Health benefits of the Half-twist pose.
- It improves the posture.
- It relieves back pains and helps prevent scoliosis and osteoporosis.
- It tones the abdominal muscles.
- It relieves stomachache and gastritis.

The Sage Twist Pose

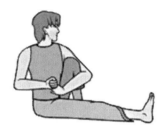

How it is done:
- From the easy mode, stretch your legs straight and hold them close to each other.
- Bend your right knee towards your chest. Keep your back straight.
- Take a deep breath. As you exhale, twist your upper body to the left. Wrap your right knee with your left hand.
- Using your hands, press the knee closer to the chest as you twist as far as you can.
- Hold the position for a few seconds. Take deep breaths.
- As you exhale, relax the hold of your left hand on your right knee and straighten your body.
- Straighten your right leg. Let it relax a little before doing the procedure with your left leg.

11. **Corpse pose.** This is usually the last pose in yoga. This aims to make the body relax before doing some stretching or yoga workouts. This is also one of the easiest poses to do.
12.

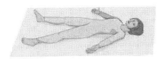

How to do it:
- Lie flat on your back on your mat.
- Stretch your arms to the sides. Spread your legs, too.
- Reach as far as you can with your hands while taking a deep breath. Slowly release your breath while relaxing the muscles in your hands.
- Rotate your feet four times in a clockwise direction then another four times in a counter clockwise position. Point your toes to the wall and stretch your legs as far as you can while taking a deep breath.
- Smile. Move your neck from side to side. Look straight to the sky. Stretch your neck up as much as possible while taking a deep breath. Slowly relax your neck as you release your breath.
- Stay in the position for 15 to 20 minutes.
- Raise your legs. Place your feet flat on the floor while still on the floor.
- Turn to the side and help yourself into a sitting position. The yoga session or routine is usually finished at this point.

Health Benefits of Corpse Pose
- It relieves back pain and other muscle pains.
- It calms the mind and relaxes the body.
- It reduces stress and alleviates insomnia.
- It strengthens your respiratory system.

Q: Do you I have to chant "om" every time I do a pose?

A: A yogi does not have to chant "om" each time he does a pose. Chanting "om" is incorporated to yoga because it helps the yogi relax and concentrate. It also helps the yogi control his breathing.

If you are not comfortable with chanting "om", you can play sounds of nature to help you relax.

CHAPTER 3:
WARM-UP ROUTINES FOR YOGA

Warm-up is necessary in every exercise. It aims to warm up the muscles to make you ready for your exercise activity. It helps protect the soft tissues from injury.

It is also essential in preparing the heart of the changes of the heartbeat and the sudden change of blood circulation. Doing an exercise without a proper warm-up workout may put stress on the heart and can be cause serious health problems or accident.

There are three ways of warming up your body before an exercise. These are the general warm-up, passive warm-up and specific warm-up.

General warm-up includes jogging, stretching and light calisthenics. Passive warm-up is warming the body using the Jacuzzi or sauna rooms. Specific warm-up includes the proper preparation needed in a specific form of exercise or practice.

This chapter will discuss the specific warm-up exercise for yoga and the steps on how to do them.

The Eye Exercise
Most yoga poses requires the eyes to look up and down or to follow the motion of the hands or feet. Thus, the eyes need to be warmed-up to avoid sudden ruptures of the eye veins or ligaments.

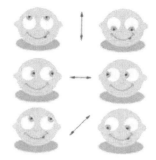

How to do it:
1. Look up and down on eight counts.
2. Look left and right on eight counts.
3. Look in the upper left and upper right on eight counts.
4. Look in the lower left and upper right on eight counts
5. Roll your eyes clockwise four times.
6. Roll your eyes counter-clockwise four times.
7. Repeat the routine two times.

Health benefits of the exercise:
- It improves the vision and helps correct eye disorders.
- It strengthens the eye muscles and alleviates eyestrains.

Face exercise

In yoga, it is not only the limbs and the body that feels the tension. The face is also subject to pressures and strains while doing the poses. Thus, it should also be warmed-up before the actual yoga practice.

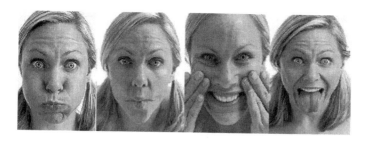

How to do it:
1. Fill your mouth with air, as much as you can, in order to make your cheek expand. Take four deep breaths. Then slowly release the air from your mouth.
2. Suck your cheek in as much as you can. Take four deep breaths and slowly release your cheeks.
3. Smile as wide as you can. Place your ring fingers on each edge of the lips and pull the skin up. Take four deep breaths. Release the edge of the lips and slowly pull the lips into a point. Point as far as you can. Take four deep breaths and slowly return your lips to its normal shape.
4. Open your mouth as wide as you can. Lift your eyebrows up as your mouth opens. Take four deep breaths. Hide your teeth with your lips and form an "o". Take four deep breaths. Smile while your teeth are hidden with your lips. Take four deep breaths. Rest your lips.
5. Pull your head back and stretch out your neck. Push your chin out as far as possible. Take four deep breaths. Pull your chin in. Take four deep breaths. Rest your chin.
6. With your head still pulled back, repeat the routine in number 3. Exhale as you straighten your head.

Neck exercises

To prepare your body from neck stretching poses required for the yoga poses, you have to warm-up your neck. Just follow the simple steps below to warm up your neck.

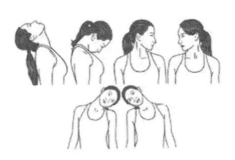

How to do it:
1. Pull your head back as far as you can. Take four deep breaths. As you exhale, pull your head down to your chest until your chin touches your chest. Take four deep breaths. Exhale as you straighten your head.
2. Twist your head from left to right on eight counts.
3. Pull your head from left to right on eight counts.
4. Rotate your neck in a clockwise direction and in a counter clockwise direction. Repeat this step three to four times.

Shoulder and Hand Exercise
The shoulders and hands receive a lot of tension during the yoga practice. A good shoulder and hand warm-up will make the poses more comfortable.

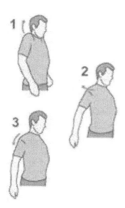

How to do it:
1. Raise your shoulders up as high as possible. Hold the position as you take deep breaths four times. On your last exhale, slowly lower the shoulders to the rest position.
2. Pull your shoulders back as far as you can. Squeeze your shoulder blades tightly. Take four deep breaths. Exhale as you return to the rest position.
3. Rotate your shoulders backwards on eight counts. Then, rotate them forward on eight counts.

4. Take a strap. Hold it on the edge. The width should be the same as your shoulders. Raise your arms up to the chest level. As you inhale, pull your hands back up as far as possible. Exhale as you return your arms to your chest. Repeat the movement four times.
5. While holding the strap, rotate your wrists on both clockwise and counterclockwise direction on eight counts.
6. Join your fingertips together. Spread your fingers as wide as possible. Join your fingers together without joining your palms.

Knee and Feet Exercise

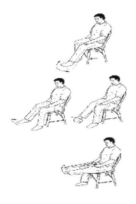

How to do it:
1. Sit on a chair. Raise one of your feet and move it from side to side. Repeat the process with the other foot.
2. Raise your foot again and rotate your ankle clockwise eight times. Then rotate it counterclockwise for eight times. Repeat the process with the other foot.
3. Take a long strap. Place your foot in the middle of the strap. Suspend your leg from the floor. Lift your leg up and down using the strap. Do this eight times. Repeat the process with the other foot.

Breathing Exercise
Breathing exercise will help open up your lungs for the tension breathings that you may get while doing yoga.

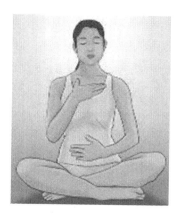

How to do this:
1. Assume the easy pose. Refer to the previous chapter.
2. Place one of your hands on your stomach and the other on your chest.
3. Take a deep breath while counting up to five. As you inhale, use your hand to push your stomach in. Hold your breath for three seconds.
4. Exhale slowly for eight counts. As you exhale, slightly push your chest in and relax the hand on the stomach.
5. Repeat the exercise at least five times.

Tip: When doing yoga poses, remember to inhale every time you stretch. Also, be sure to exhale as you bend.

After you are done with these simple yoga-specific exercises, you are now ready take on proper routines.

CHAPTER 4:
BASIC ROUTINES

The Sun and Moon Salutations
The Sun and the Moon Salutation are the most basic yoga routines. They are devotional routines to the sun and the moon, but most yogis use these routine as daily morning and night yoga routines because of their simplicity.

These routines combine the breathing exercise and the regular yoga exercise. The daily practice of these routines will bring many health and therapeutic benefits to the yogi.

The Sun Salutation

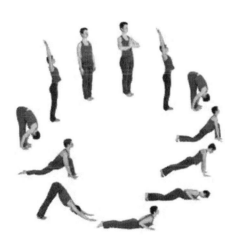

How to do it:
The sun salutation begins and ends with the mountain pose.
1. Do the whole mountain pose.
2. Then, do the forward bend.
   To do the forward bend: Bend forward from the mountain position. Reach for your ankle and let your chest rest on your thighs. If you find it difficult as a beginner, you can hold on to your calves instead. Take

four deep breaths using the breathing exercise method.
3. Proceed to the Lunge Pose.
To do the lunge pose: From the forward bend, slip your right foot to the back. Your instep and knees should touch the floor. Your shoulders, left knee, left heel, and hands should be aligned together perpendicular to the floor. Take four deep breaths using the breathing exercise method.
4. Proceed to the plank position.
To do the plank position: From the lunge position, slip your left foot beside your right foot. You will be assuming a dog position. Raise your hips and take on a downward facing dog position. Refer to chapter 2 to know how to do it.
Then move your shoulders up to align with your hand. Lower your buttocks and hips as you move your shoulders. You will be assuming a basic push-up pose.
5. Continue to the 8-limb position.
To do the 8-limb position: From the plank position, lower your body onto the floor. Raise your hips and tailbone. Breathe.
6. Do the cobra pose.
To do the cobra pose: From the previous position, lower your hips and tailbone towards the floor. Slowly bend your back upward as high as possible.
7. Return to the downward facing dog position. From the cobra pose, lower the upper body to the floor again. Raise your hips up and assume the downward-facing dog position.
8. Do the lunge position again, but your left leg should be the one at the back.
9. Slip your left leg to the front and join it with the right leg. Slowly raise your hip and tailbone and assume the forward bend.
The last step is a reverse mountain pose. You will start from the raised-arm pose and continue to the

prayer pose. You will end up in the mountain pose again.
10. Repeat the salutation three times.

The Moon Salutations

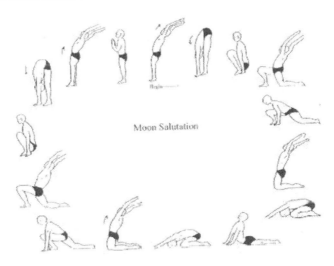

Moon Salutation

How to do it:
Like the sun salute, the moon salute starts and ends with the mountain pose. Here are the complete steps:
1. Do the mountain pose.
2. Do the forward bend pose.
3. From the forward bend pose, drop to the squat pose.
   To do the squat pose: Without moving your hands and feet, lower your buttocks. Your buttocks should touch the ankle of your feet.
4. Do the half lunge pose.
   To do the half-lunge pose: Slip your right foot to the back. Lower your knee on the floor. Your body and your knee should be aligned. The knee and the feet shall be parallel to the floor.
   As you inhale, slowly raise your hand over to your head. Lower your hands back onto the floor.
5. Slip your foot further and do the full lunge pose.

6. As you inhale, assume a kneeling pose or the kneeling mountain pose. Take a deep breath and raise your hands above your head again.
7. As you exhale, rest with the child's pose. Hold the position for a few seconds.
8. Slip your body forward. Straighten your legs and assume a cobra pose. Hold the position as long as you can.
9. Rest with the child's pose again.
10. Do the kneel pose.
11. Stretch your left foot to do a full lunge pose.
12. Pull your left foot closer to do a half-lunge pose.
13. Pull your left foot to join the right foot and assume the squat position.
14. Slowly raise your buttocks to shift into the forward bend pose.
15. While inhaling, raise your upper body to return to the mountain pose.

According to some yoga experts, three complete routines of sun salutation every morning and three complete routines of moon salutation in the evening are equivalent to an hour of jogging and other calisthenics. Each salutation usually takes only 3 to 5 minutes. That would sum up to only 20 to 30 minutes of workout a day.

Health Benefits of Sun and Moon Salutation
Doing the sun and moon salutation daily has many healing benefits. Aside from the specific healing effects of each pose, the routine is said to:
1. Strengthen abdominal muscles or flattens the belly. The routines are good ways of losing the extra flabs in the hip and stomach area.
2. It sharpens the memory and improves the nervous system.
3. It helps detoxify the body, expelling toxins and carbon dioxide.

4. It corrects hormonal imbalances, prevents goiter, and alleviates menstrual disorders.
5. Prevents alopecia, hair fall, and graying of hair.
6. It improves longevity.
7. It aids in weight loss.

Basic Yoga Routine
Below is a very basic standing, sitting, and lying routine which you can use as an alternative or supplementary routine for the sun and moon salutation. It uses the most basic poses discussed in Chapter Two.

PART 1: Basic Standing Routine
How to do this:
1. Stand in the mountain pose. Do the raising the arms pose. Stay on the pose for 15 seconds.
2. Slowly lower your hands to your chest and assume the prayer pose.
3. Take a deep breath and slowly raise your praying hands above your head again while simultaneously placing your left foot on your right thigh. You will be assuming the tree pose. Hold the posture for a minute.
4. Slowly lower your hands and your thighs. Assume the prayer pose again.
5. Repeat step 3 using your right foot and your left thigh.
6. Repeat step 4.
7. From the prayer pose, slide your left foot to the back and take on the basic warrior pose. Spread your hands at shoulder level and do 6-8 twists.
8. Assume the prayer pose again.
9. Repeat step 7 using your right foot.
10. After the last twist, do not return to the prayer pose but take on the basic triangle pose. Hold a triangle pose for each side for 15 to 20 seconds.
11. Return to the prayer pose and proceed to doing the mountain pose.
12. Do the forward bend pose.

Part 2: The Basic Sitting Routine

13. From the forward bend, slowly lower your buttocks and take on the squat pose.
14. From the squat pose, shift to the easy pose. Do 5 breathing exercise while in the easy pose.
15. From the easy pose, do the half-twist pose. Hold the half-twist pose for each leg for 15 to 20 seconds. Do two sets of half-twist pose.
16. Stretch your legs together and do the sitting forward bend. Exhale as you bend.
17. Raise your torso and do the sage twist. Hold each twist for 15 to 20 seconds. Do two sets of sage twists.
18. After the last sage twist, repeat step 16. Straighten your back.
19. Curl your knees a little and using your arms as support, slowly lie on the floor and assume the basic corpse pose.

Part 3: The Basic Lying Routine

20. While on the corpse pose, do the leg raising pose. Raise your left leg. Your leg and your body should be perpendicular with each other. Breathe. Hold the position for 10 to 15 seconds. Repeat the procedure with your right leg.
21. Return to the corpse pose.
22. Simultaneously raise both your legs together. Hold the position for 10 to 15 seconds. Then do the scissors motion with your legs for eight counts. After the scissors motion, continue to raise your legs together.
23. Slowly pull your knees towards your chest. Wrap your hands on your shin and press your curled legs tightly to your chest. This is known as the gas release pose. Do not be surprise if your gas is really released.
24. Release your legs return to corpse pose.
25. Curl your legs and assume the basic bridge pose. Do the bridge pose for 15 to 20 seconds. Repeat the pose three times.

26. Return to the basic corpse pose. Hide your hand behind your butt. Raise your chest and pull your head back. This is called the Fish pose. Hold the position for 10 to 15 seconds. Repeat the pose three times.
27. Return to the basic corpse pose and do the whole corpse poses.
28. Rest for a minute or two. Turn to your side and assume a sitting position and proceed to doing the mountain pose. You have completed the routine.

If you aim to lose weight, use this as a supplementary routine for the sun and moon salutations.

As you continue to practice this basic routine, your body is expected to become more flexible. Soon, you will be able to do advanced poses.

Q: Where is the ideal place to do yoga routines?

A: The ideal place to do yoga routines is the studio where yoga classes are held. The humidity of the room is pre-set by the teacher to make you comfortable. The floor is made to be clean and safe for you when assuming floor or lying poses.

But if you are doing yoga on your own, any place with flat floor is ideal to practice your routines. Just make sure that the humidity of the place is comfortable for you and the air is clean.
You can also do yoga at the park or in your backyard so you can be close to nature.

CHAPTER 5: PREPARING FOR THE ADVANCED YOGA POSES

Some of the powerful and therapeutic poses in yoga are so advanced that preparations are needed before doing them. In this chapter, we will discuss some advance yoga poses, how they are done and how you can prepare yourself to achieve the poses.

The Plough Pose
The plough pose or the "plow" pose is a difficult pose. Without proper guidance and proper preparation, it can also become dangerous.

The pose aims to relieve chronic neck pains. It also strengthens the kidneys, the spine, the gall bladder, heart, and the liver.

It also cures bad posture.

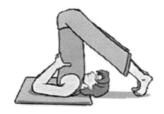

How to do it:
1. Lie on the floor or on the mat. Hold your feet together. Place your hands above your head, palms facing upward.

2. Raise your legs together. Your leg and upper body should be in a 90-degree angle.
3. Slowly raise your hips and push your legs down towards your chest. Bring your legs over to your head. Your toes should touch the floor.
4. Keep your back straight. Your chin should be pressed on your chest. Slip your hands to your sides and use them to support your back.
5. Hold the position for at least 15 seconds.
6. One by one, bring your legs back to the floor and slowly straighten your back and assume the corpse pose.

How to prepare your body for the plow pose:
1. Lie down near the wall. Raise your legs up the wall. Move your body closer to the wall. Your legs and your buttocks should be pressed on the wall.
2. Slowly raise one of your legs and bring it towards your face. You do not have to touch the floor or your face yet. Just feel the contractions of your hips. Hold the position for 15 seconds. Repeat the process with your other leg. Do three sets for this exercise.
3. Place your legs back to the wall. Join them together and bring them towards your face. Hold the position for 15 seconds.
4. Place your legs back to the wall. Slowly raise your hips and elevate your buttocks. Press your raised buttocks on the wall.
5. Repeat step 3. Try to push your legs deeper.
6. Repeat step 4 but raising your hips and buttocks an inch or two higher. Then repeat step 3.

Tips for the beginner:
You are not expected to touch the floor on your first preparation exercise. With continued practice of the preparation exercise, you will soon be able to touch the floor. Be patient.

It will also help if you will have somebody to assist you. Let another person hold your legs as you bend them forward. That way, you can control the fall of your legs towards your face.

The Shoulder Stand

One of the difficult pose of yoga is the shoulder stand. In this pose, your whole body will be supported by your shoulders and neck only.

This pose is intended to strengthen your shoulders and your back. It also tones your core muscles.

This pose also helps the internal organs, especially the thyroid glands. It stimulate the growth hormone and correct hormonal imbalances. It also improves the blood circulation. It also alleviates stress and insomnia.

Some studies show that the shoulder stand also helps the woman become fertile and prepare their body for childbearing and childbirth. This is because the pose strengthens the pelvis, which is the core muscle that aids in pregnancy and childbirth.

There are two ways of doing this pose. The direct shoulder stand pose, wherein your directly assume the pose, and the indirect shoulder stand pose, which you assume after doing the plough pose.

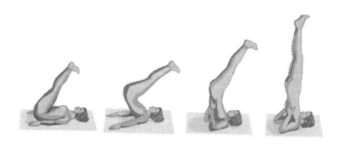

How to do it the direct way:
1. Lie flat on your mat or on the floor and assume the corpse pose.
2. Bring your hands to the side. Raise your legs up.
3. Lift your hips higher and push your feet over to your head. Your shoulders, biceps and elbows should support you.
4. Hold your hips and push your back further. As you push your back, slowly pull your legs back to align with your back.
5. Once your back and your legs are aligned, hold the position for 15 seconds.
6. Curl your knees. Using your hand as a guide, slowly pull your body back to the floor or the mat.
7. End with the corpse pose.

How to do it the indirect way:
1. Do the plough pose.
2. From the plough pose, raise your legs up and let it align with your back.
3. Hold the position for 15 seconds. Then fall back to the mat in the same process as the plough pose.

How to prepare your body for the plow pose:
1. Lie down near the wall. Slowly bring your legs up to the wall. Move your body closer to the wall. Your legs and your buttocks should be pressed on the wall.
2. Slowly pull raise the height of your legs by lifting your hips off the floor. Continue to increase the height of your legs as you lift your hips. Use the wall to support your legs and your hips.
3. When you reach your limit, hold the position for 15 seconds. Slowly lower your body back to your original position.
4. Repeat the process again but increase the height of your legs until you reach the straight shoulder stand with the support of the wall.

Tips for the beginner:
Make sure that your shoulders and elbows are not slipping from the position. Collapsing from a shoulder stand can damage some vertebrae in your body which can be dangerous.

Do the shoulder stand with a partner or an instructor so they can render better support and control during your practice.

The Backbend pose
The backbend pose is another difficult pose. In this pose, your legs are pulled over to your head while bending your back.

This pose helps increas your ability to focus. It is a good exercise for the brain. It sharpens the memory. It relieves stress, insomnia and anxieties. It boosts your confidence. It also strengthens the heart, rib cage, and the spine. It also helps relieve constipation and other digestive problems.

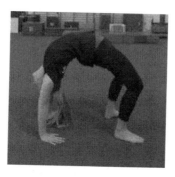

How it is done:
1. Assume the basic bridge pose.
2. Place your hands to the sides of your head and bring your elbows towards the cieling.
3. Slowly push your hips up to do the bridge pose.
4. Using your hands, push your head and upper body up so your whole body is suspended to the air. Only your feet and your hands will be supporting your body.

5. Hold the position as long as you can.
6. To get up from the pose, slowly lower your hips back to the floor. Then lower your upper body back to the floor, too. Roll to the side. Assume a sitting position before standing up. Another alternative is to give your upper body a push forward.

How to prepare your body for a backbend:
1. Take a short stool. Sit on the edge of the stool. Slowly lower your upper body. place your hands on the floor. Your elbow should be facing the ceiling and your fingertips should be pointing towards your heel.
2. Slowly move your hips away from the stool. Let your back rest on the stool while your head is pulled back to the floor. Your hips should be aligned to your chest.
3. Push your whole body up and away from the stool. Hold the position as long as you can. Rest your back to stool again. Repeat the process but make sure to keep the body suspended on the air longer each time.

Soon, it would be easy for you to hold your position even without touching the stool. Continue to use the stool for support until you are confident enough to do the bend without the stool.

The Head-to-feet Backbend
The head-to-feet backbend is a variety of backbend. This is more difficult than the regular backbend. This is also called the scorpion pose.

Like the regular backbend, it strengthens the brain and the heart. It also improves focus, alleviate stress, anxiety and insomnia. This variety however makes the core muscles more powerful than the regular backbend.

There are two ways to do this pose. There is the indirect way which continues from the regular backbend and the direct backbend, wherein the yogi directly performs the pose.

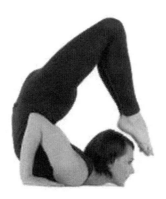

How to do the direct backbend:
1. Lie face down on the mat or on the floor.
2. Place your hands on the sides. Curl your elbows. Your elbows should be towards the ceiling.
3. Raise your upper body as you raise your legs towards your head.
4. Let your chest support your body. Stretch your hands and reach for your feet. Pull your feet towards your head. Your can rest your feet to your head if you can do so.
5. Place your hands back to the sides and resume its original position.
6. Hold the pose for as long as you can.
7. To get down from the pose, return your legs, one by one, to the floor.

How to do the indirect backbend:
1. Do the regular back bend.
2. Slowly, roll your chest towards the floor or the mat.
3. As your chest gets close to the floor, lift your legs, one by one from the floor.
4. Hold the pose for as long as you can.
5. To get down from the pose, just continue to roll your chest and hips towards the floor until your legs can be placed to the floor.

How to prepare for the Head-to-Feet Backbend:
If you are doing the indirect backbend, use the preparation for the regular back bend as the first part. Then crawl down the stool and let your chest touch the floor. Your thigh should now rest on the stool. Hold the position.

Keep practicing the backbend until you are confident enough to take away the stool.

If your are doing the direct backbend, you should try to use straps. Tie a strap on each of your ankle. Then assume the basic position. Reach out for the straps. Using the straps, pull your legs towards your head. Pull as far as you can.

Once you have reached your limit, hold the position for as long as you can. Keep repeating the steps until your legs can easily reach your head.

Now that you know some advanced poses, you can now incorporate them into your basic yoga routines to achieve better health.

CHAPTER 6:
THE YOGA DIET

Yoga is not only about posture and poses. It consists of the total healing of the body. A healthy diet is an essential part of the healing of the mind body and spirit. Thus, a yogi should also know the food he should eat and should avoid to achieve a calm mind and stress-free state.

According to some yoga experts, there are three kinds of healthy food.

The first are the healthy foods that stimulate and relax your mind. These are the organic, natural, unprocessed and easy to digest. Examples of these are whole grains, mung or lentil beans and clarified butter.

The second are healthy foods that disturb your mind because it may give you an addiction or withdrawal symptoms. Examples of these are chocolates and coffee. Though these foods have some healthy benefits for your body, however, too much and too often consumption of these can disturb your mind.

The third are the healthy foods that make your mind dull. These foods, though healthy, tend to make your mind lazy or lethargic. Examples of these are spices such as garlic and onions. Red meat is also proven to make the mind and the body lazy, heavy and lethargic.

The Recommended Diet
The original recommended diet for yoga is called the Sattvic diet. It is composed of eating rice, lentils, clarified butter and vegetables. The diet is also low of lethargic spices such as garlic and onions and disturbing spices such as hot peppers.

Sattvic diet is eating the foods in their natural state, as much as possible.

However, many experts believe that the diet cannot suffice the physical activities of yoga. Since the muscles and the bones receive tensions during poses, the yogi diet should include foods that are high in calcium and high in protein. This is why many yoga instructors are suggesting that yogis should observe a vegetarian diet instead, which are still low of lethargic and disturbing spices.

Here is the list of the food to eat and the food to avoid during the yoga practice:

Food to Eat	*Food to avoid*
Apples and pears Oatmeal Watermelons Raisins and prunes Almonds Dried apricots Mung beans or lentils All vegetables except onion and garlic Fresh Organic Soy Milk Soy products Sweet spices like cinnamon and basil Molasses, raw honey and organic maple syrup Banana Berries	Red Meat Onions and garlics White flour products Products with Refined Sugar Processed foods Canned vegetables Fried foods Animal fats Plants and animals that were genetically engineered and non-organic Soda drinks, coffee and chocolates

Frequently asked questions about the Yogi Diet
Are fish and chicken not allowed when doing yoga?

Fish and chicken are not prohibited when doing yoga. It is only highly recommended to avoid them.

When doing yoga, the foods that should be eaten are those that are easy to digest. Since fish and chicken are a bit heavy on the stomach, yogis are advised to avoid them.

Should I drink herbal teas while doing yoga?
Herbal teas are highly recommended because they keep the body hydrated. They also help in detoxifying the body. If you are not used to drinking herbal teas, you can drink vegetable juices instead.

Herbal teas are recommended to be taken after the yoga class. This is because yoga poses stimulate the detoxifying process of the body. Many yogis claim that they tend to do big dumps after yoga sessions. If you drink herbal teas before the yoga class, it may speed up the detoxifying process and may cause you to leave the session to go to the bathroom.

Would it be bad to milk while doing yoga?
Milk is high in calcium and protein and should be in your yoga diet. Organic animal milk, especially cow's milk, are allowed in the yoga diet but should be consumed in appropriate portions.

PREVIEW OF 'ZEN FOR BEGINNERS'

CHAPTER 01: ZEN LIFESTYLE

Zen is a Japanese term for 'meditation'. Zen monks were devoted to live their lives in concentration and mindfulness. They are devoted to serve others on a daily basis. You may probably never become a Zen monk, but there are ways to adopt their 'mindful' living.

Is it really possible to be mindful of our life and our surroundings? Can you really achieve happiness by simply taking notice of what's happening around you? Yes, you can do both things with Zen.

Zen lifestyle is a way to become more aware of your connection to the world and other inhabitants. One of the most quoted Zen monks, Thich Nhat Hanh, said, "We have more possibilities available in each moment than we realize." If you come to think of it, you'll realize that it's certainly true.

Now, if you want to learn more about the guiding principles of Zen lifestyle, read the list below. Bear in mind that these principles are not 'religious practices'. You can apply them in your life no matter what kind of lifestyle standard or religious beliefs you have.

1. Do things one step at a time. One of the best guiding principles of Zen lifestyle is preventing multitasking. In the world of high technology, people are becoming more excited to do more than they can manage at a

time. There's a Zen proverb that goes, "When walking, walk. When eating, eat." That explains a lot.
2. Whatever you're doing, do it slowly and deliberately. The other common problem that people are facing today is rushing through things from time to time. It's simply because they want to accomplish more things at a time, but the truth is if you take time in doing a certain thing, you'll get better results. This is because when you're not in a rush, you'll be able to focus on the task at hand and see clearly what needs to be done.
3. Do less. Zen monks are not lazy, but they don't also have a list of hundreds of tasks to do in a day. So that gives them more time to concentrate on whatever they chose to do. If you start doing fewer things in your life, you'll see that it would be easier for you to follow guidelines number 1 and 2.
4. Allow breaks between your tasks. In this principle, you will be able to learn how to manage your schedule. Don't imprison yourself in a tight schedule. Take a break after and before doing each task. This way, you'll have time to relax your mind and prepare yourself for another task at hand.
5. Finish your work. Don't proceed to another task when you are not yet finished with the one at hand. When you did your work completely, you'll be able to be more focused on your next task.
6. Develop rituals. Ritual is a way of giving importance to your work or to anything that you are doing, including eating and running. You are not required to do Zen rituals – you can create your own. Create a ritual for food preparation, for eating, for going to exercise, and for everything that you do daily.
7. Assign a specific time for each task that you want to accomplish for the day. You should set a particular time for eating, for taking a shower, for dressing up,

and more. You can do this for your daily routines and your work activities.

8. Spend some time in sitting. One of the most important things for Zen monks is their time for meditation, which is mostly done by sitting in a quiet place. The act of meditation is a practice to be present. You can do this in any way you like, as long as you achieve inner peace and calmness.

9. Practice smiling and serving others. Zen monks spend their lives in serving other people, from both inside and outside the monastery. Serving others will teach you how to be humble and it will help you realize that you are not just a selfish creature. You can start serving within your family circle and friends. Also, smiling can improve the lives of those who are around you.

10. Make cooking and cleaning a part of your meditation. Cleaning and cooking can sometimes become boring chores because they seem like just a part of your daily routine. But when you turn them into a part of your meditation session, you'll become more mindful in doing them and achieve better results.

11. Focus on what's necessary. You are not required to live exactly like a Zen monk, who is contented with basic clothing, shelter, and tools. But somehow, you must learn how to live only with what's really important for you. Living with all the unnecessary things can only clutter your life and lead you to careless lifestyle.

12. Live in a simple way. This is somewhat related to guideline number 11. If you are living only with the necessities, then you could achieve a simple lifestyle. Essential things may differ in every individual. There is no particular law regarding to what should be important for all of us. It's up to you to think about these things and learn to keep them and let go of those that are not important.

If you can follow these 12 simple guidelines, you will be able to enjoy your life even better. Don't forget what Thich Nhat Hanh said: "Smile, breathe, and go slowly."

TIPS TO PRACTICE ZEN LIFESTYLE

The guidelines above summarized the core concept of Zen lifestyle. Many people are very much intrigued with the lifestyle because it sounds promising. However, beginners may always find it hard to adhere to the guidelines simply because they have grown too old to change their old ways.

Don't worry! There are 6 simple tips that you can learn in order to easily apply the guidelines of simple, mindful living.

1. Don't compare yourself with others. When you compare yourself, your lifestyle, your career, your education, your appearance, or your intelligence with others, you will end up suffering. You will always find someone who is better than you in many ways. But when you stop comparing yourself with others, you'll see the brighter side of the picture. You'll become more respectful and appreciative of others. Hence, you'll be able to be grateful in your own uniqueness.
2. Stop judging other people. This is opposite of comparing, because in judging, you are deemed to see the worst in others. You feel like you are better than most and you are likely to refuse any kind of help and lesson from other people who are concerned with your welfare.
3. Stop worrying for the things that are not yet happening. Worry is a product of fear and the need to control situations. When you are constantly worried about things, you are not only suffering by yourself but you are also creating heavy burden in other people who are surrounding you.
4. Stop blaming others. Blaming is one way of protecting yourself from being judged. It is also easier to blame

rather than accept responsibility for the mistakes you've committed. When you blame others, you cannot look deeper into the situation to find a solution to the problem. So instead of putting the blame on others, try to be reasonable and see what went wrong and be responsible enough to resolve the problem.
5. Don't compete with others. Competition is fun when you're just playing for the game and not for the results. But when you begin to be concerned about the results, you will begin to increase your ego and do everything to prevent others from getting ahead of you. Just be competitive in a way of improving yourself, not in being indifferent to others.
6. Learn to laugh. The easiest way of living is not to take things too seriously. There are certain things in our lives that require focus, diligence, and attention but those should not stop you from having fun. Additionally, when you are enjoying what you do, you will hardly feel bad about your life.

These tips sound obvious and you hear them every day but it's about time to be determined in implementing them in your life. Knowing something is knowledge but you'll develop wisdom when you start to properly apply the things that you've learned.

CHAPTER 2:
BUILDING YOUR CHARACTER

In this chapter, we will dig deeper into effective ways on how you can totally apply simplicity in your life and how to combat many negative situations that will come your way in the future.

First, let's talk about how you can live in a peaceful, contented, and happy way.

Here are the best tips that you can follow:

1. Study the things or people that are more important to you. What is it that you really want to do? Who are the people that matter most to you? List down (on a sheet of paper) the things that you want to do, the people that you want to spend more time with, and the goals that you'd like to achieve in the future.
2. Take time to examine your short-term and long-term commitments. Many people suffer from many problems because their schedules are always full. You can't possibly do all the things that you have committed to do. Therefore, you must accept the fact that you can't do everything. Eliminate the commitments that don't matter and stick with those that are most important.
3. Aside from commitments (for family, friends, or work), we also have lists of 'things-to-do' for the day or for the week. Now that you have eliminated some commitments from your schedule, you must proceed to eliminating some unimportant things from your to-do list.
4. Set aside days when you don't have to do anything. Forget all about your responsibilities, take time to relax and enjoy the day by yourself.

5. Find mentors and inspirations. Look for people who can inspire you. Read books that can motivate you.

By following these 5 simple steps, you will be ready to embrace the simplicity of the Zen lifestyle. Enjoy!

DEALING WITH OBSTACLES

Now, let's talk about how to deal with obstacles in life. There will always be problems and struggles that will come your way. No matter what you are trying to achieve in life, there will be moments when you might want to give up.

When you have decided to change your lifestyle, it is also expected that you will face difficulty. It's not really that easy since you are changing not only your ways of living but also your perspective about things that surround you. These obstacles are dangerous since they can stop you from achieving your goals or slow you down.

Here are a few tips that you can apply when facing these obstacles:

1. Learn to identify the obstacles. It's not easy to realize that a certain situation or individual that is trying to hinder you from achieving your goals. Some people who are close to you (e.g. spouse or trusted friends) can say things that may cause you heartbreak. Determine the difference between realistic criticisms and humiliating insults. Listen closely to what they say and observe your own reaction. If the words seem to discourage you and make you feel like quitting, then those people might be your roadblocks.
2. Examine if they have valid points. As discussed in number 1, you need to know if these people are being realistic. They might have a good reason for their negative feedback. But if their negativity is not valid, consider number 3.

3. Block out all the negativity that they are injecting in your mind. Detractors have a way of effectively transferring their negative thoughts into your mind. You'll suddenly feel doubtful and it will result to crashing the foundation of your plans and goals in life. Don't think about them again and again. Push the negativity and replace them with positive thoughts. Don't allow them to rule over you.
4. Bear in mind that there will always be obstacles and people will always have different opinions. You can't do anything to prevent them but you can practice how to ignore them. You don't have to push them away from your life, but learn how to simply smile at them when they are talking. Their words won't have any effect in you if you chose to ignore them.
5. Learn how to make them approve your plan. There are times that the detractor is a person who is very close to you and you can't simply ignore him. Instead of arguing, help this person realize the importance of your goal. Let him know that you also have doubts but that shouldn't stop you from believing that you can achieve it someday. Let him know about the positive benefits that you'll get once you achieve these goals.
6. Learn how to laugh with your detractors. Many people can feel uncomfortable when you suddenly take a leap of change. They may probably tease you and make fun of you. This is the only way they can do to deal with this change. In order to make them feel at ease with your new plans, laugh with them when they tease you. This will make it easier for them to take things lightly and realize that it's not really such a big deal.
7. Prepare your counterarguments. Some people simply talk negatively because they are misinformed. Prepare yourself to educate them about the change in you. Do it in a positive way so as to make the conversation enlightening. You may or may not be

able to change their minds. But either way, you were able to clear your points to them.
8. Take refuge in the knowledge that you are doing something good. You can't always win other people and make them entertain your beliefs. Sometimes all you can do is ignore them. Just bear in mind that in the end, you will enjoy the benefits of your hard work and that is the prize for ignoring your detractors.

Always remember that detractors are simply a part of the journey that you have to overcome. There will always be obstacles but if you don't give up, you will be successful in the end.

OVERCOMING DEPRESSION
Depression robs people of their happiness. It makes us feel insecure and weak. It can cause a lot of trouble in life including inability to work properly, broken relationships, and feelings of emptiness to name a few.

Traditionally, you can undergo therapies that can help you bring back your self-esteem and courage. However, there are also other practical ways that won't cost a dime and can make you feel better in the long run.

Here are some tips:

1. Get out of your comfort zone. That means you should get out of your house and expose yourself to sunlight. Sunlight aids in keeping your internal clock working properly.
2. Get enough sleep at night. Turn your lights off when you go to bed. Engage yourself in calming activities before your sleep. Read a book or take a warm bath. Get to bed early. When you are depressed, you will always feel tired and a tired body needs a good night rest.

3. Socialize with people you love. It's not easy to surround yourself with people when you don't feel like it but you have to do it. You don't actually have to force yourself in deep conversations. Just be present. When you are always surrounded with people, you will eventually feel less isolated.
4. Watch your thoughts. Be mindful of the things that come to your mind. Stop every negative thought that wanders in your mind and keep your thoughts positive and happy. It will take some time to work this out but if you do this constantly, you will eventually turn it into a habit.
5. Play lively music. Music is a great therapy. Allow yourself to move with the beat of music. It helps to release your emotions.

Just like the other habits that you are trying to learn in Zen lifestyle, you don't need to do this all at once. Pick out one habit at a time and do it until you feel better.

CHAPTER 3:
ZEN WORKING LIFESTYLE

Every one of us dreams to become successful someday. Whatever field of work we are trying to pursue, we all want to reach a certain point in our lives when we can finally savor the fruits of our labor.

In that case, we need to form successful habits to achieve our goals. In order to be successful, you must not only rely on your working capabilities but you must also work in building successful habits in your personal life.

Og Mandino shared in his book, *The Greatest Salesman in the World*, one of the most powerful concepts about developing a habit. He explained that in order to turn something into habit, he would do the same thing continuously for 30 days. It sounds easy, but a lot of us could hardly make it to 20 days in trying to form a new habit. After skipping, we would soon revert to our old pattern and begin to forget all about the habit that we wanted to develop.

But Zen lifestyle offers excellent strategies on how you could implement this new development in your life.

1. Be committed. The first thing that you need to do is to commit yourself on doing the new habit for 30 days.
2. Develop a morning habit of reading a mantra silently. You can create something on your own or you can find suggestions from Zen master's books.
3. Develop a midday habit of reading the mantra again. Remember to read it silently.
4. In the evening, read the mantra again but aloud this time.
5. Create a habit chart to track your progress. Everyday put a mark on the chart to see what day you are on. Don't miss a day. If you missed it, start all over again.

6. Plan for future habits. Once you've achieved this first habit (mantra reading), start other habits that you want to develop. It could be something that you want to do in your home or at work. Don't forget to create a chart for each habit that you are trying to develop.
7. Create personal motivational notes and post them on places where you can see them often. This way, you'll be able to be motivated to accomplish your goal for the month.
8. Celebrate for yourself every time you accomplished your goal. (See chapter for simple ways of rewarding yourself.)

Optimism is generally the key to become more successful in achieving your new goals. Whenever you form new habits, you are molding your own character that can help you build your confidence in your career.

Check out the rest of Zen for Beginners on Amazon.
http://www.amazon.com/dp/B00MBFE3IC

CHECK OUT MY OTHER BOOKS

Below you'll find some of my other popular books that are popular on Amazon and Kindle as well. Simply click on the links below to check them out. Alternatively, you can visit my author page on Amazon to see other work done by me.

1. *Buddhism for Beginners: A Practical Guide to Embrace Buddhism Into Your Life*
   http://www.amazon.com/dp/B00P2S5NYI
2. *Zen For Beginners: Achieve Today Your Happiness and Inner Peace with Zen Buddhism*
   http://www.amazon.com/dp/B00MBFE3IC
3. *Kundalini for Beginners: Awaken Your Kundalini Within To Heal Your Body Naturally*
   http://www.amazon.com/dp/B00PLMT0H6
4. *Reiki for Beginners: Master the Ancient Art of Reiki to Heal Yourself and Increase Your Energy*
   http://www.amazon.com/dp/B00QPDKB0K
5. *Chakras for Beginners: A Practical Guide To Radiate Energy, To Heal and Balance Yourself Through the Power of Chakras*
   http://www.amazon.com/dp/B00QP7SUEK
6. *Mindfulness For Beginners: A Practical Guide To Awakening and Finding Peace In Your Life*
   http://www.amazon.com/dp/B00RH36DIG
7. *Feng Shui For Beginners: Master The Art of Feng Shui To Bring More Balance, Harmony and Energy Flow*
   http://www.amazon.com/dp/B00RQPFGQU

CONCLUSION

Thank you again for downloading this book!

We hope this book was able to enlighten you about what Yoga is and encourage you to try this practice in order to achieve a calm mind and stress-free living.

As this book had shown you, some poses in this book are difficult and are a bit dangerous. I suggest that upon reading this book, you should enroll in a yoga class so your knowledge about the poses will be reinforced by a proper yoga instructor.

Finally, if you enjoyed this book, then I'd like to ask you for a favor, would you be kind enough to leave a review for this book on Amazon? It'd be greatly appreciated!

Please leave a review for this book on Amazon!

Thank you and good luck!
Alexander Yamashita

Made in the USA
San Bernardino, CA
31 August 2016